HEART DISEASE DIET COOKBOOK FOR VEGANS

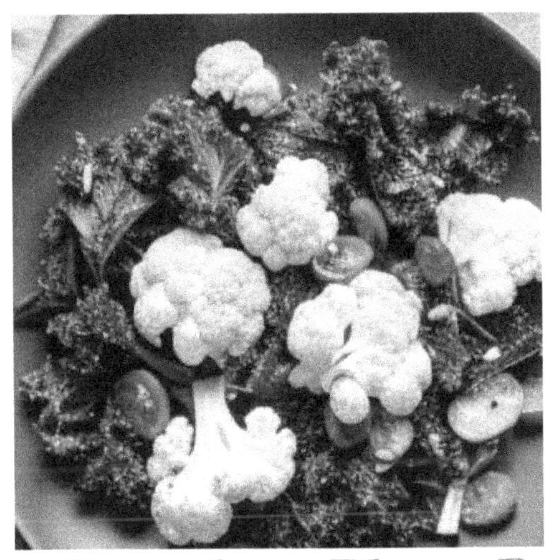

The Complete Plant-Based Recipes Guide to Healthy Heart

Jessica Murray

Dear Reader,

Thank you for the purchase. I hope you enjoy and love it, would you consider dropping an honest feedback/review, I will appreciate that and you can contact me using JessicaMurrayDietHelp@gmail.com if you have any questions, I will gladly respond

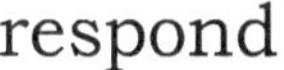

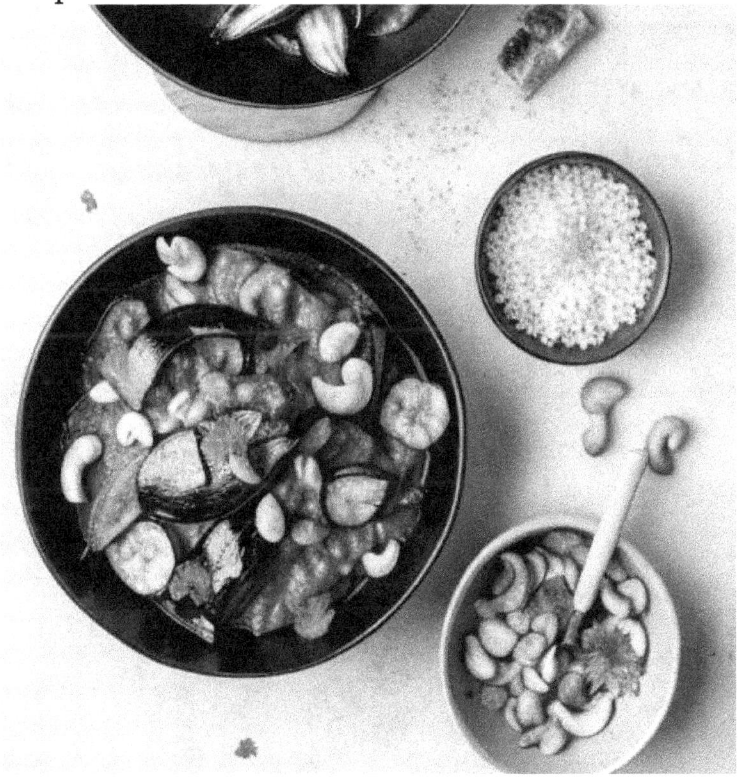

Table of Contents

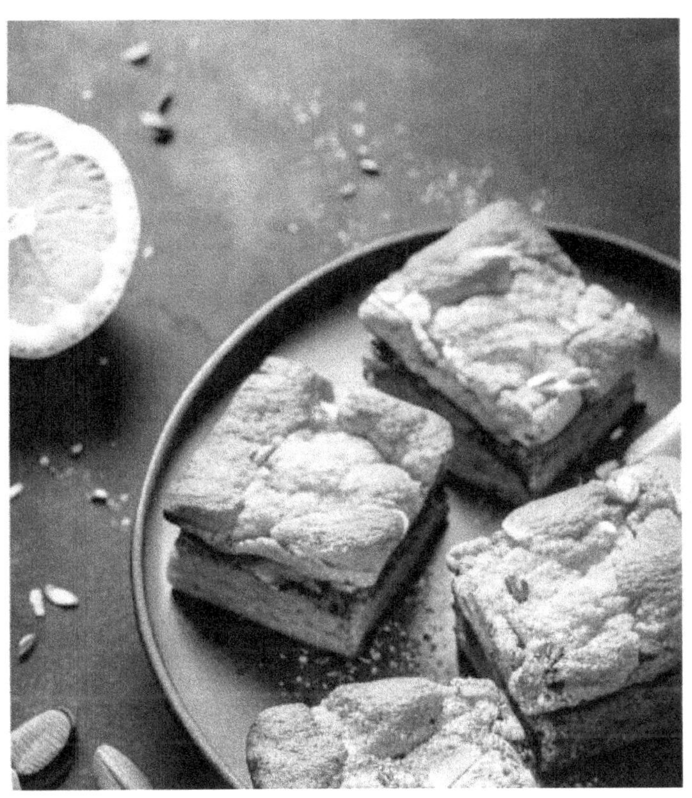

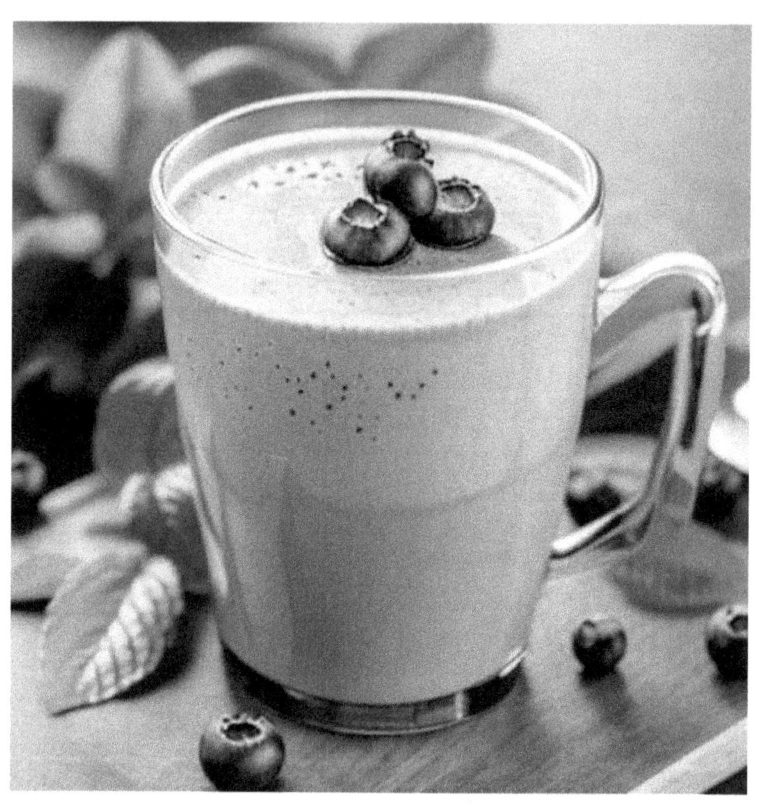

INTRODUCTION

John had a heart condition that had been present for more than ten years. He was prescribed a variety of medications, and he was advised to switch to a heart-healthier diet. He had tried a variety of food regimens, but he had never exactly found one that was effective for him. He was a vegan, but he discovered that none of the vegan meals he had tested offered the health benefits he was hoping for.

His doctor then advised him to try the Vegan Heart Disease Cookbook in particular. He was first dubious, but after following the recipes for a few weeks, he began to see improvements in his health. He had more energy, felt less out of breath while going about his regular business, and was losing weight. The outcomes astounded him!

After following the recipes in this cookbook for a few months, John's heart health had significantly improved. His energy levels were through the ceiling, his blood pressure and cholesterol statistics had normalized, and he was continuing to lose weight. He had a complete transformation! The Vegan Heart Disease Cookbook had positively altered John's life. He was able to rely less on prescription drugs and more on the natural curative properties of food. He was incredibly delighted to have found this cookbook because his health was better than it had ever been. He was able to maintain a vegan diet while significantly enhancing his heart health, which was something he had never thought was possible.

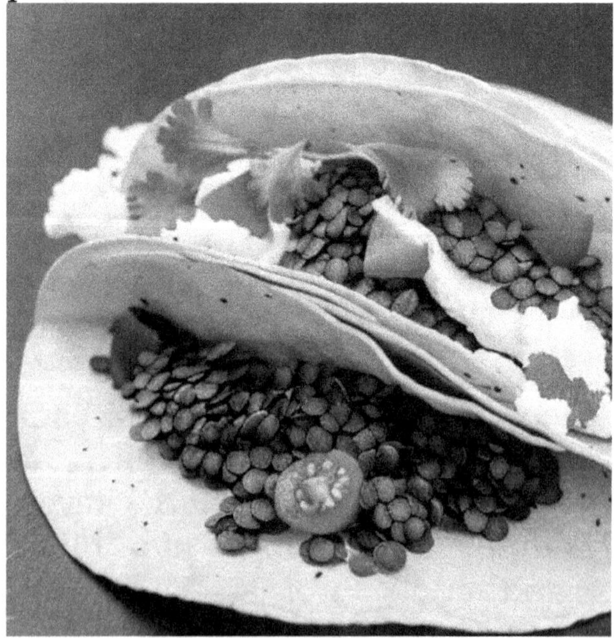

CHAPTER 1

BREAKFAST RECIPES
Banana Nut Overnight Oats

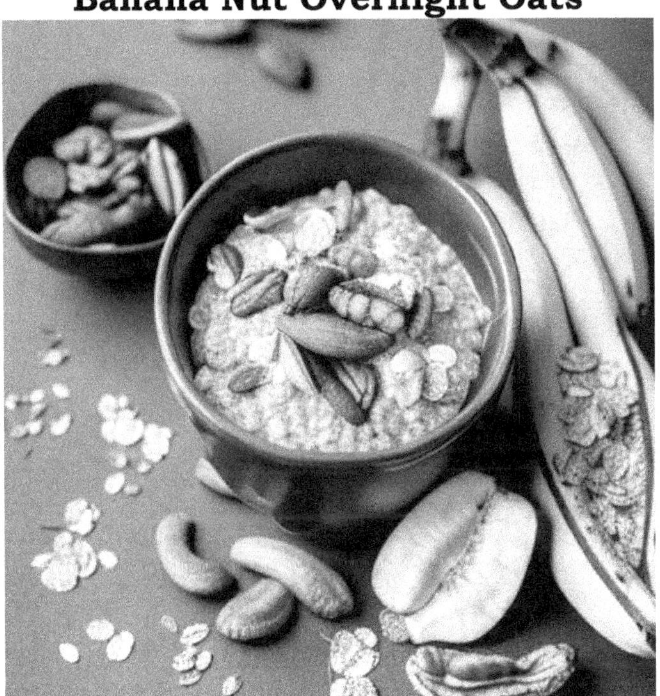

Ingredients:

- 1 cup rolled oats
- 1 cup plant-based milk,
- 2 tablespoons chia seeds,
- 2 tablespoons almond butter, and
- 3 tablespoons chopped walnuts or pecans
- 1 sliced banana

Instructions:

- Oats, chia seeds, and plant-based milk should be combined in a medium bowl
- Add almond butter and blend by stirring.
- Put the mixture in the refrigerator for the night.
- Add the walnuts or pecans in the morning, then sprinkle the banana slices on top
- Enjoy!

Baked Mushroom and Asparagus Frittata

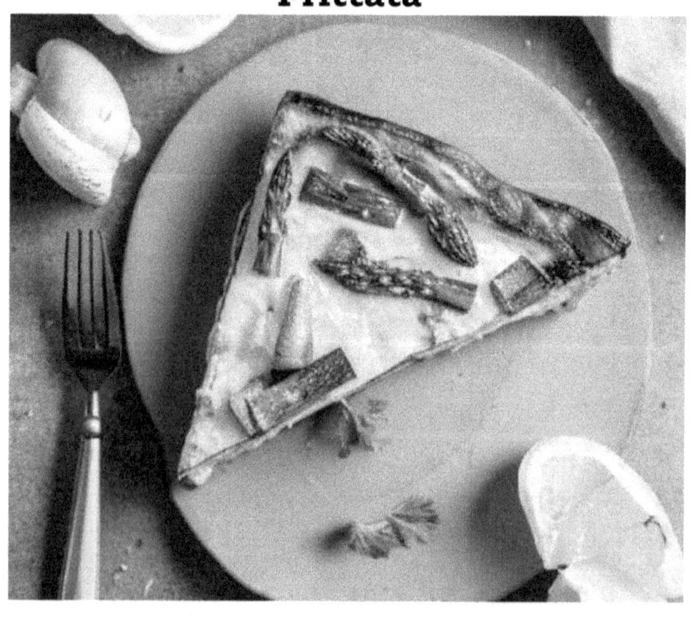

Ingredients:
- 1 tablespoon olive oil
- 1/2 chopped onion, and 2 minced garlic cloves.
- 8 ounces of sliced button mushrooms
- 2 cups chopped asparagus
- 6 eggs
- 2 tsp. nutritional yeast
- black pepper and sea salt.

Instructions:
- Set the oven to 375 degrees.
- In a large skillet set over medium heat, warm the olive oil.
- Add the onions and garlic and simmer for 3 minutes, or until softened.
- Include the mushrooms and simmer for 5 minutes, or until golden brown.
- Add the asparagus and simmer for an additional 2 minutes, or until tender.
- Whisk eggs in a sizable bowl.
- The eggs should be combined with the cooked veggies and nutritional yeast after being added.

- Fill a 9-inch baking dish with the mixture after seasoning it with salt and pepper.
- Bake for 20 to 25 minutes, or until the eggs are fully cooked, in the preheated oven.
- Enjoy!

Avocado Toast with Roasted Tomatoes

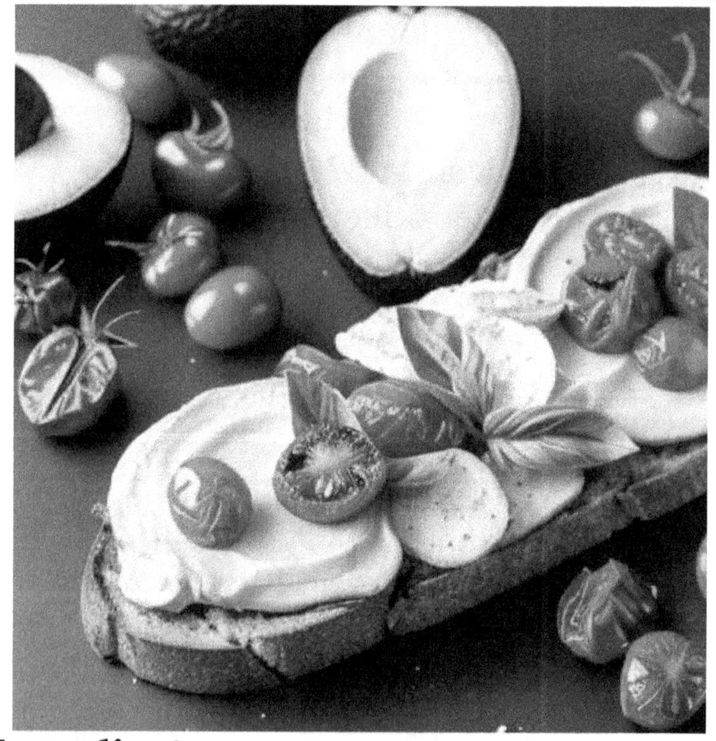

Ingredients:
- two large tomatoes that have been cut into wedges.

- 2 slices of whole grain bread;
- 1/2 mashed avocado
- 1 tablespoon olive oil2 tablespoons of cilantro, chopped finely
- black pepper and sea salt.

Instructions:

- The oven should be preheated to 375°F.
- Arrange the tomato wedges on a parchment-lined baking sheet.
- Sprinkle salt and pepper on top of the tomatoes before adding the olive oil.
- Bake for 15–20 minutes, or until the tomatoes are softly roasted and golden brown, in the preheated oven.
- Slices of whole-grain bread are toasted in the toaster.
- Top the toast slices with the roasted tomato wedges after spreading the mashed avocado over them.
- Add some cilantro and salt and pepper to taste
- Enjoy!

Almond Butter and Jam Toast

Ingredients:

- 2 slices of wholegrain bread
- 2 tablespoons of almond butter.

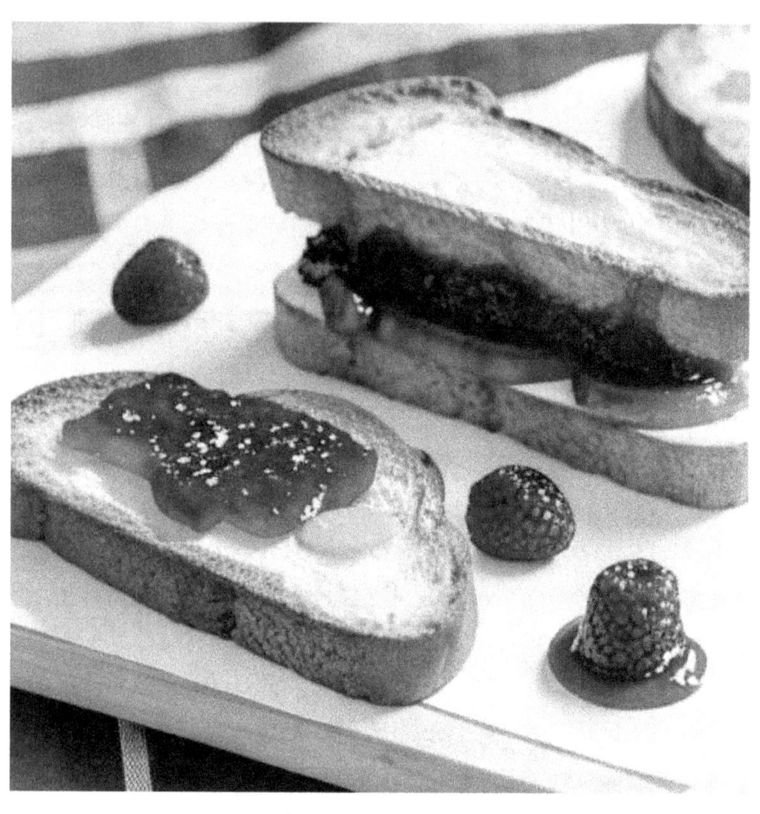

Instructions:

- In the toaster, toast the slices of whole-grain bread.
- One slice should have jam on it, while the other should have almond butter.
- Almond butter side down, stack the slices of bread, and cut each one in half.

- Dispense and savor!

Buckwheat Waffles

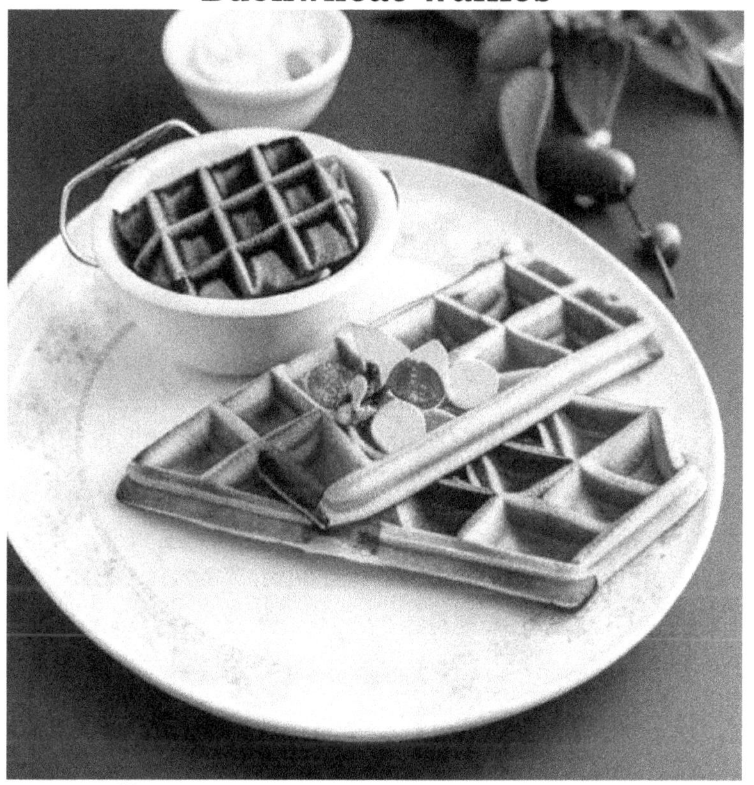

Ingredients:

- 1 cup buckwheat flour
- 1 teaspoon baking powder
- 1 cup plant-based milk
- 2 tablespoons vegetable oil
- 1/4 teaspoon sea salt,
- 1 teaspoon pure maple syrup

Instructions:

- Combine the buckwheat flour, baking soda, and salt in a medium bowl.
- Combine the plant-based milk, oil, and maple syrup in a separate bowl.
- Just blend the dry ingredients with the wet components after adding them.
- Waffle iron on high heat with a light oil coating
- Pour the batter into the waffle maker that has been warmed, and cook for 5 minutes or until crispy and golden brown.
- Enjoy! Serve with the toppings of your choosing!

CHAPTER 2

LUNCH RECIPES
Charred Cauliflower and Kale Salad

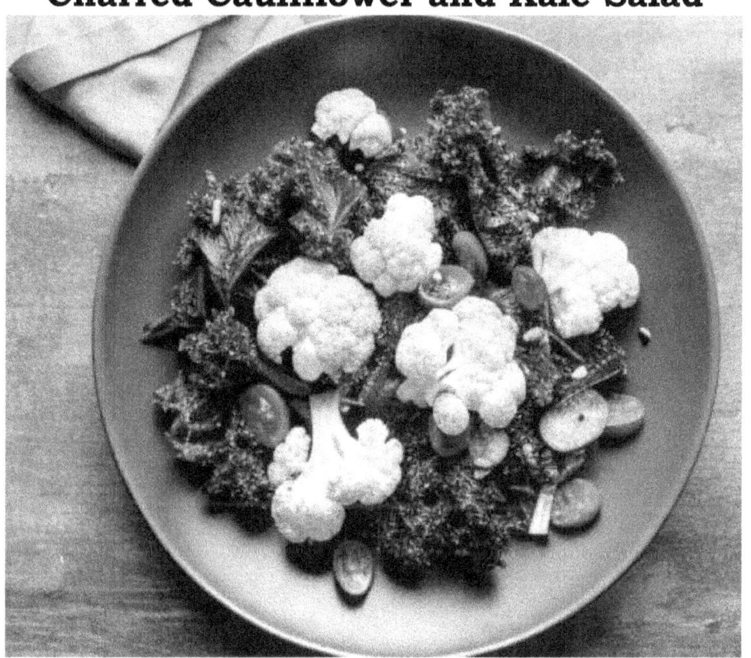

Ingredients:

- 1 cauliflower head, cut into florets
- oil of olive
- 3 cups of roughly chopped kale, salt, and pepper 1/4 cup of slivered almonds
- currants, 1/4 cup
- Lemon juice, two tablespoons

Instructions:

- Start by setting your oven to 375°F.
- On a baking sheet, arrange the cauliflower florets and sprinkle with olive oil. Salt and pepper the food, then roast it for 25 minutes.
- blend the kale, almonds, currants, and lemon juice in a sizable bowl and stir to blend while the cauliflower roasts.
- After the cauliflower has finished cooking, add it to the kale in the bowl and stir to incorporate. Serve hot.

Avocado Chickpea Wraps

Ingredients:

- 2 ripe avocados, peeled and mashed;
- 1 15-ounce can of washed and drained chickpeas
- 2 minced garlic cloves.
- 1 teaspoon each of smoked paprika and ground cumin
- Chile powder, 1/4 teaspoon
- To taste, salt and pepper
- 4 whole wheat tortillas

Instructions:

- In a bowl, combine the chickpeas and avocado by mashing them together.
- Include the cumin, smoked paprika, chili powder, salt, and pepper along with the minced garlic. Assemble by combining.
- After the tortillas have been spread with the mixture, roll them up. Serve.

Roasted Vegetable Bowls

Ingredients:

- 1 sweet potato, diced
- 1 bell pepper, seeded
- 1 red onion
- 1 cup cooked quinoa
- and 1 cup cooked black beans.
- Olive oil, two tablespoons

- To taste, salt & pepper

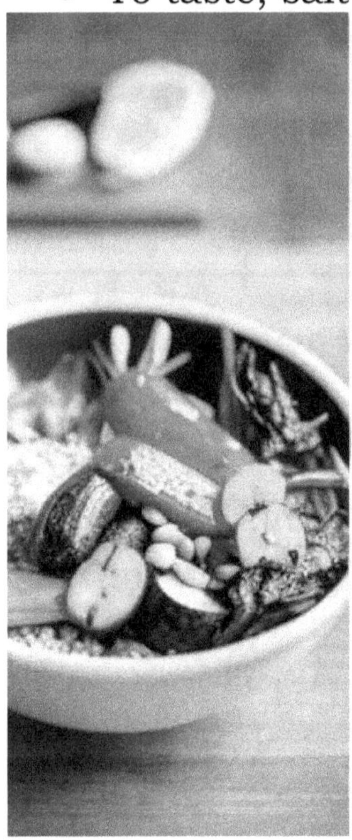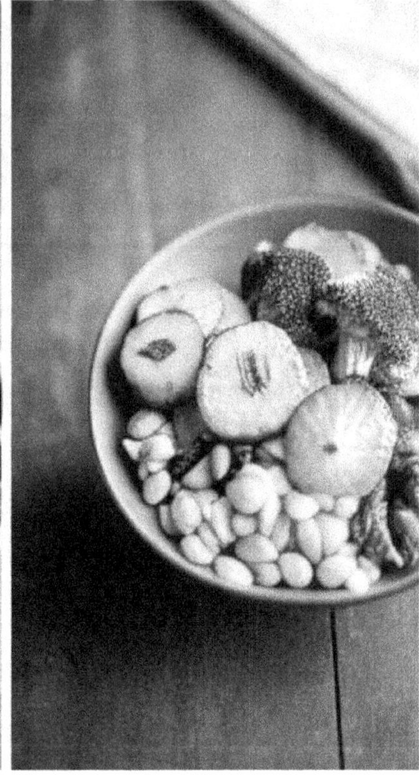

Instructions:

- Start by setting your oven to 375°F. Place the red onion, bell pepper, and sweet potato in a single layer on a baking sheet and sprinkle with olive oil. Add salt and pepper to taste. For 20 minutes, roast.

- After the vegetables have finished cooking, divide them among the four dishes.
- Equally distribute the quinoa and black beans among the dishes, then stir everything together. Serve hot.

Fennel, Apple and Walnut Salad

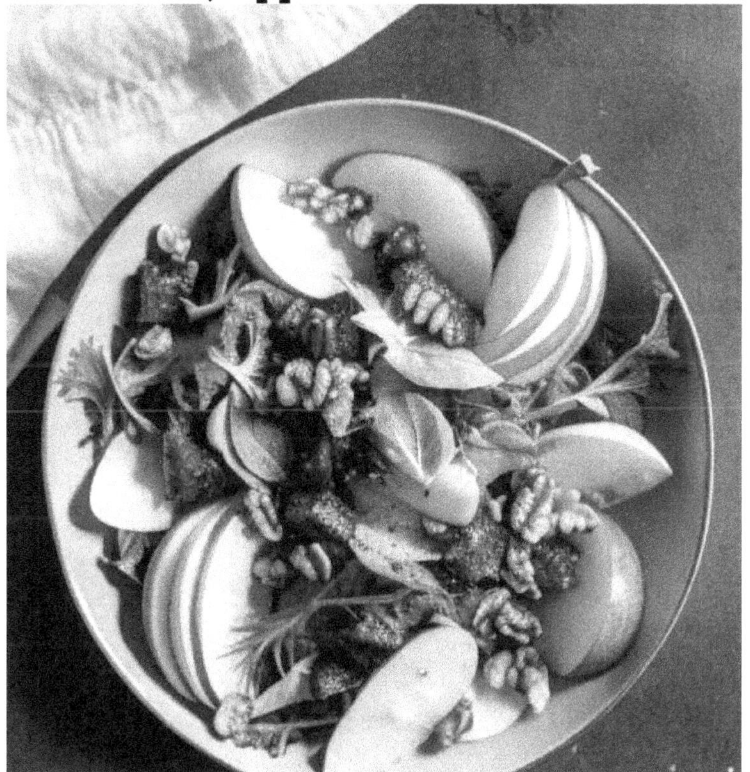

Ingredients:
- 1 thinly sliced bulb of fennel

- 1 cored and diced apple; 1/4 cup of chopped walnuts.
- 1/4 cup of feta cheese in crumbles
- two teaspoons of lemon juice and one tablespoon of olive oil
- To taste, salt & pepper

Instructions:

- Combine the fennel, apple, walnuts, and feta in a big bowl.
- Combine the olive oil, lemon juice, salt, and pepper in a small bowl.
- Drizzle the salad with the dressing and toss to mix. Offer cold.

Lentil Tacos

Ingredients:

- one tablespoon of olive oil, two minced cloves of garlic
- and one small diced onion
- a single teaspoon of chili powder
- 1 teaspoon of cumin powder
- 8 mini taco shells
- Plus salt and pepper to taste
- 1/2 cup of cheese, shredded

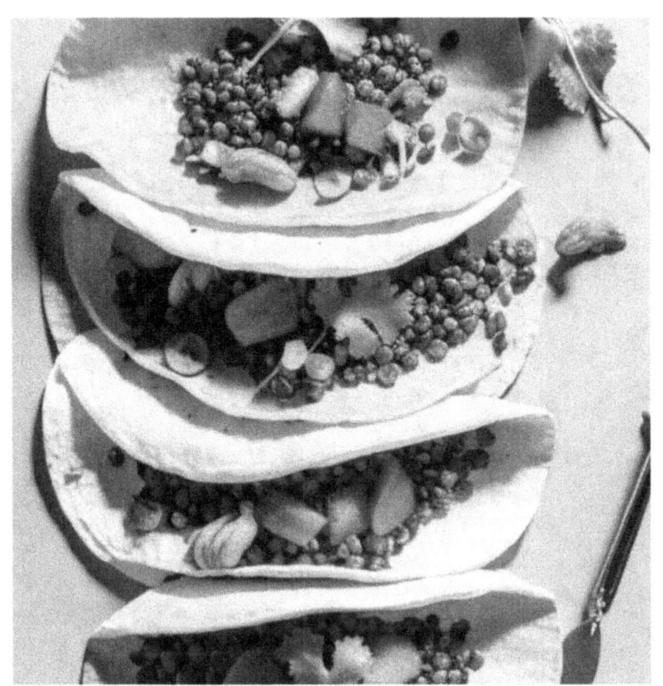

Instructions:

- Heating a large skillet over a medium flame, pour in the olive oil.
- Include the onion and cook it until it softens. Once the garlic has been added, sauté for 1 minute.
- Once the lentils are heated through, add the cumin, chili powder, salt, and pepper.
- Add cheese on top of each taco shell after adding a tablespoon of the lentil mixture. Serve.

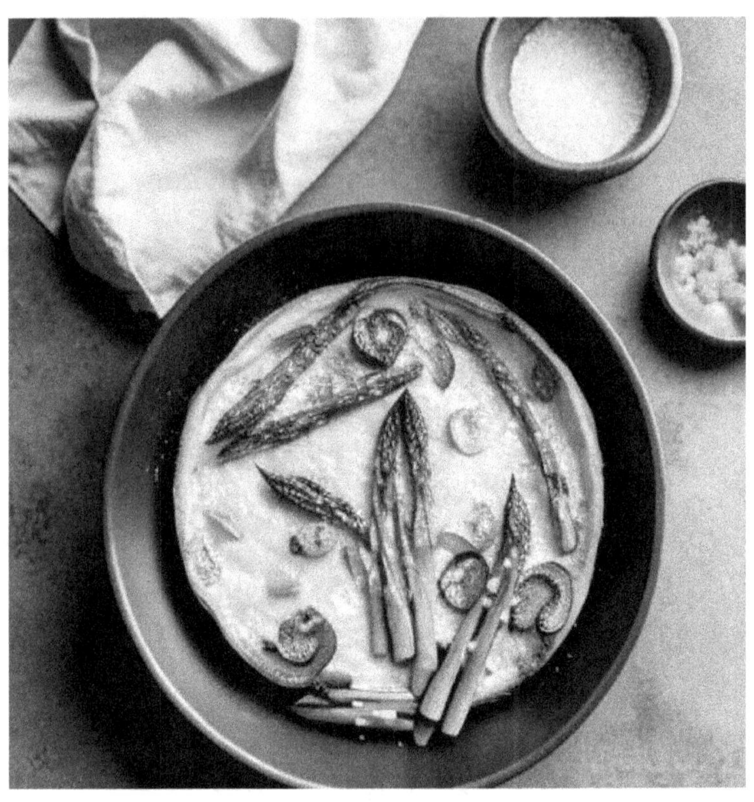

CHAPTER 3

DINNER RECIPES
Quinoa Stuffed Peppers

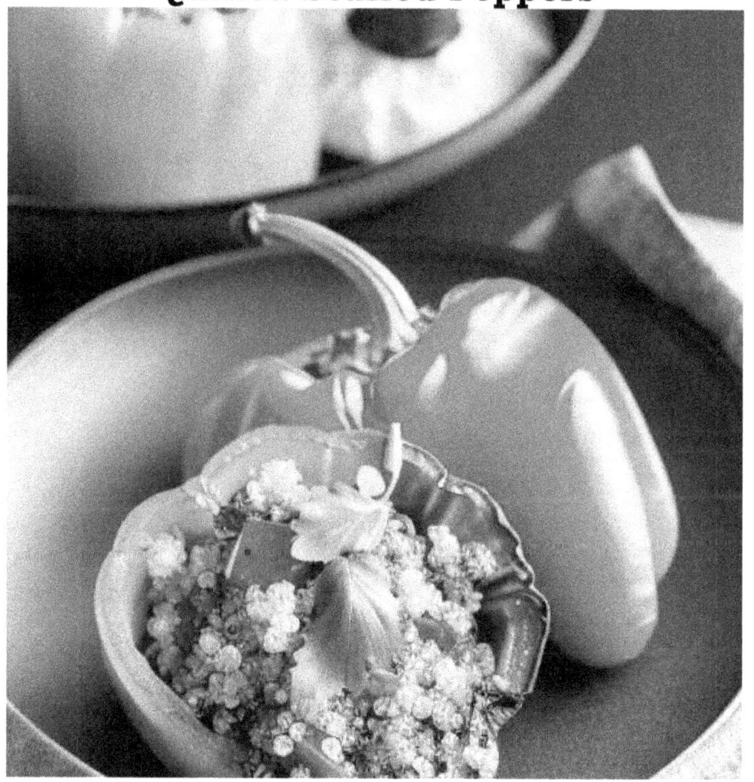

Ingredients:

- 1 cup quinoa and 4 bell peppers
- 1 tablespoon of olive oil and 1 teaspoon of garlic powder
- 1 cup of diced onion, 1 cup of diced carrots

- 1 cup of veggie broth; taste-tested salt and pepper

Instructions:

- Set the oven to 350 degrees Fahrenheit.
- Halve the bell peppers and scoop out the seeds.
- Set the oil in a large skillet over medium-high heat.
- Add the onion and carrots. Cook until softened, for 5 to 7 minutes
- Include the quinoa and heat until just faintly toasted.
- Stir in the garlic powder and vegetable broth, then bring to a simmer.
- Allow the quinoa to simmer for 10 to 15 minutes, or until it is cooked and the liquid has been absorbed.
- Stuff the quinoa mixture inside the bell peppers.
- To make the peppers soft, bake them for 20 to 30 minutes.
- After adding salt and pepper, serve the dish warm.

Super Green Pesto Pasta

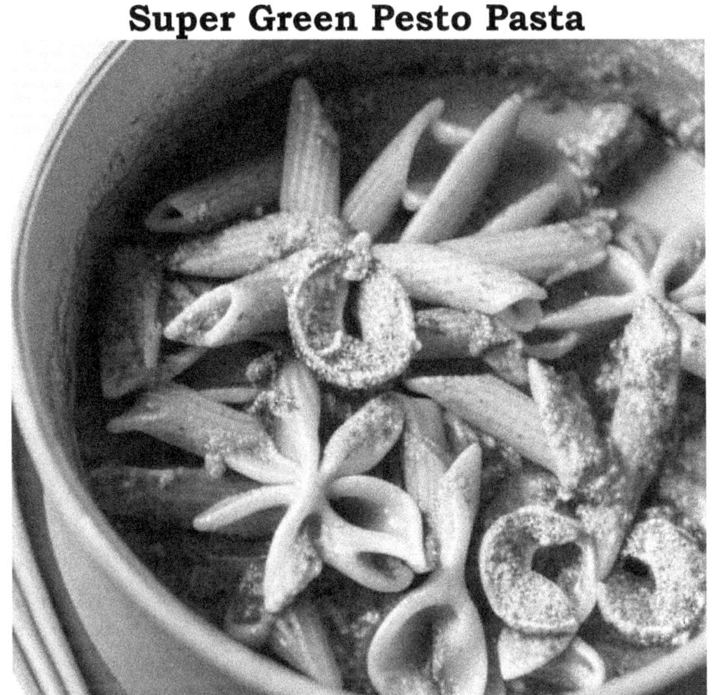

Ingredients:

- 2 tablespoons olive oil, 2 minced garlic cloves,
- and 8 Ounces gluten-free pasta.
- two cups of baby spinach;
- two cups of kale
- 3/3 cup uncooked cashews
- 1/4 teaspoon each of salt and pepper;

- 1/4 cup nutritional yeast; and 1 lemon's juice

Instructions:

- Start by heating up a saucepan of salted water to a boil. The pasta should be prepared as directed on the packaging.
- In a big skillet over medium-high heat, warm the oil. Cook for 1-2 minutes after adding the garlic.
- Include the kale and spinach and blend. Cook the spinach and kale until they are wilted.
- In a food processor, combine the cashews, nutritional yeast, salt, pepper, and lemon juice.
- Stir the pesto into the skillet while adding it.
- Stir the cooked pasta into the pan after adding it.
- Present warmly and savor.

Roasted Eggplant and Cashew Curry

Ingredients:

- two large eggplants, diced;
- two tablespoons olive oil; one teaspoon each of ground cumin,

ground coriander, and garam masala;

- 1 coconut milk can
- Cashews, 1/2 cup1/4 cup finely chopped cilantro; 1 teaspoon each of salt and pepper

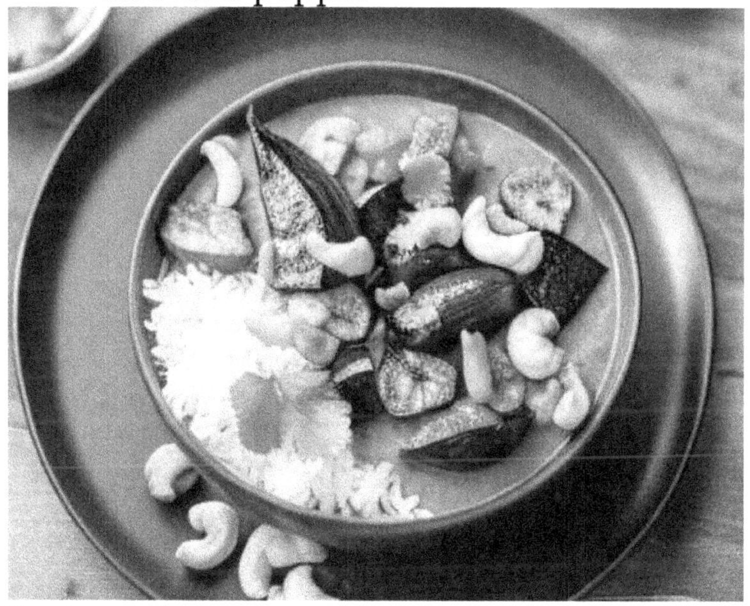

Instructions:

- Set the oven's temperature to 400 F.
- Spread some olive oil on a baking sheet and add the diced eggplant.
- Add garam masala, cumin, and coriander.

- Bake the eggplants for 20 to 30 minutes, stirring halfway through, or until they are brown and soft.
- Combine the coconut milk, cashews, and roasted eggplant in a sizable pot over medium heat.
- Bring to a simmer, lower the heat, and cook for ten to fifteen minutes.
- Add the cilantro and season with salt and pepper.
- Present warmly and savor.

Broccoli and Sweet Potato Fritters

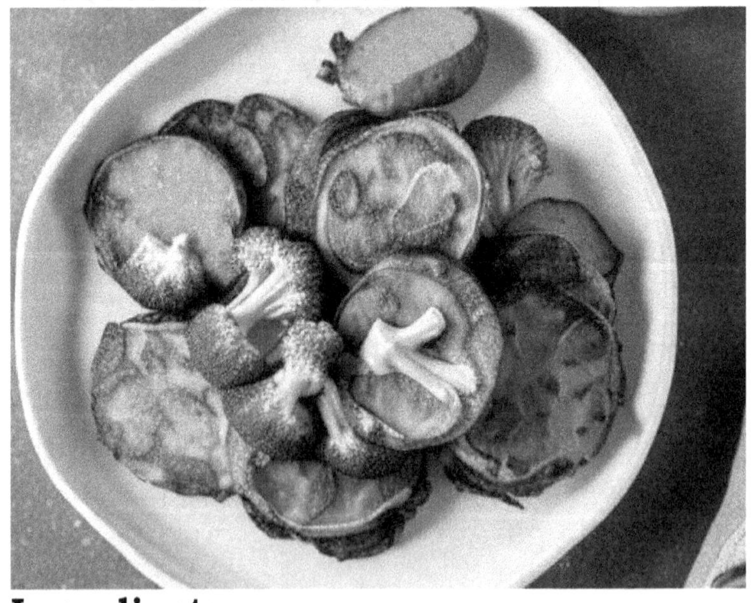

Ingredients:

- 1 cup cooked and pureed sweet potatoes
- 1/2 cup chopped onion; 1 cup cooked and chopped broccoli; 1/2 cup gluten-free flour
- One teaspoon of garlic powder
- A half teaspoon of baking powder2 teaspoons of flax meal
- Water, 2 tablespoons
- To taste, add salt and pepper.

Instructions:
- Combine the sweet potatoes, broccoli, onion, flour, garlic powder, and baking powder in a medium bowl.
- Combine the flax meal and water in a small basin and set aside for five minutes.
- Combine the flax and broccoli combination thoroughly.
- Add oil to a big skillet that is already hot over medium-high heat.
- Scoop out patties from the mixture and place them in the skillet.
- Cook until golden on each side for three to four minutes.

- Add salt and pepper to the dish as it is served heated.

Grilled Portobello Mushrooms

Ingredients:

- Three substantial portobello mushrooms
- 2 tablespoons of extra virgin olive oil
- 2 minced garlic cloves
- 2 tablespoons low-sodium soy sauce
- 2 teaspoons balsamic vinegar
- One tablespoon dried basil
- To taste, add salt and pepper.

Instructions:

- Turn the grill's heat up to medium-high.
- Wash and dry the portobello mushrooms.
- Combine the basil, soy sauce, balsamic vinegar, garlic, and olive oil in a small bowl.
- Use the mixture to brush the mushrooms.
- After the mushrooms have been placed on the grill, cook them for 5-7 minutes, flipping once.
- Add salt and pepper, then serve.

CHAPTER 4

DESSERTS RECIPES
Raw Trio Bars

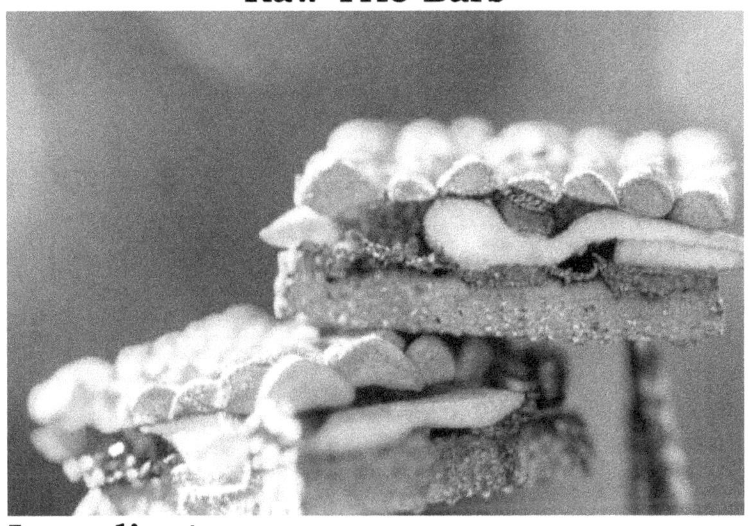

Ingredients:

- 1 cup chopped raw pecans
- 1 cup chopped raw almonds 1 cup chopped dates
- 1/2 teaspoon ground cinnamon
- 1/3 cup almond butter
- One-fourth teaspoon of Himalayan salt

Instructions:

- Pecans, almonds, and dates should be pulsed in a food processor until they are coarsely minced but not fully ground up.

- Add the almond butter, cinnamon, and salt to the mixture after you've transferred it to a bowl.
- Everything should be combined until a thick dough develops.
- Place the dough on a baking sheet that has been lined with parchment paper, and shape it into a rectangle by pressing it down with your hands.
- After roughly 30 minutes of freezing, cut the bars into bars.

Vegan Matcha Cheesecake

Ingredients:

- 1/4 cup almond milk and 1 package of extra-firm silken tofu.
- 2 teaspoons melted coconut oil
- Matcha powder, 2 tablespoons
- two tablespoons each of agave nectar, corn-starch, vanilla extract, and
- two tablespoons each of lemon juice.

Instructions:

- Set the oven to 350 degrees. A 9-inch spring form pan should be lined with parchment paper.

- In a high-speed blender, puree the silken tofu, almond milk, coconut oil, matcha powder, agave nectar, corn-starch, vanilla extract, and lemon juice until thoroughly combined.
- Bake for 25 to 30 minutes after pouring the mixture into the spring-form pan. 30 minutes to cool.
- Serve after being chilled for at least 4 hours.

Banana-Strawberry Ice Cream

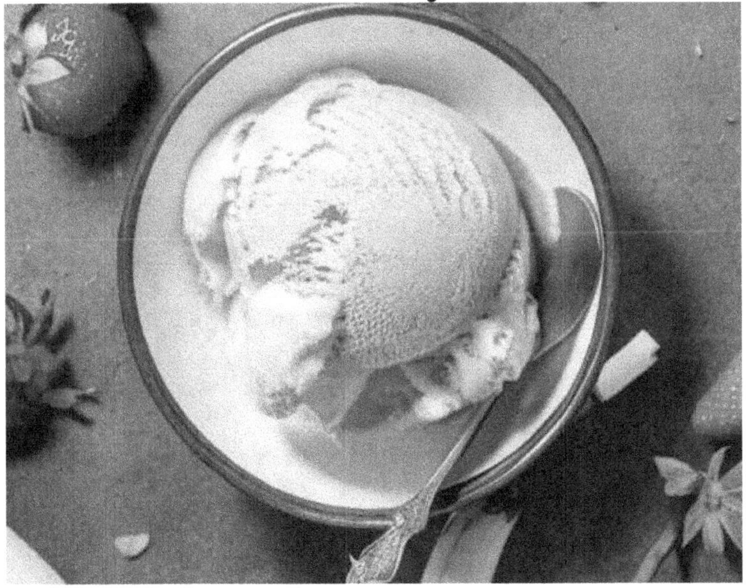

Ingredients:

- two frozen, ripe bananas
- 2 cups strawberries, frozen

- A half cup of almond milk

Instructions:

- The components should be combined in a food processor
- Pulse just enough to mix. Blend the ingredients until they are smooth and creamy after cleaning the food processor's sides.
- Before serving, transfer the mixture to an airtight container and freeze for at least 4 hours.

Coconut-Lemon Blondies

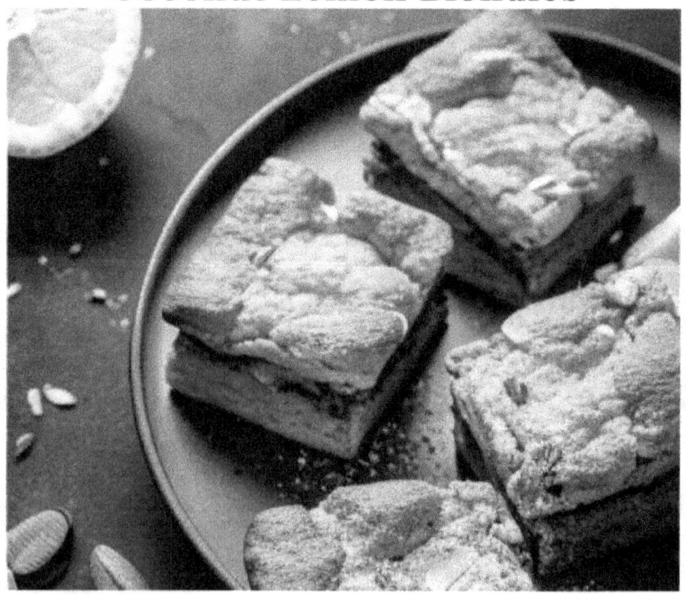

Ingredients:

- 2 tablespoons of ground flaxseed,

- 1/2 cup of melted coconut oil,
- 1/4 cup of coconut sugar, 2 teaspoons of lemon zest,
- and 1 teaspoon of vanilla flavour.
- 1/2 teaspoon baking powder
- 1 cup all-purpose flour
- One-fourth teaspoon baking soda
- salt, 1/4 teaspoon

Instructions:

- Set the oven to 350 degrees. Butter an 8-inch baking dish.
- Combine the flaxseed, coconut sugar, coconut oil, lemon zest, and vanilla extract in a medium bowl.
- Sift the flour, baking soda, baking powder, and salt in a separate basin.
- Mix the components until incorporated after adding the dry elements gradually to the wet ones.
- Bake the mixture for 25–30 minutes, or until a toothpick inserted in the centre comes out clean. Transfer the batter to the prepared baking pan. Prior to serving, cool

Chia Seed Pudding

Ingredients:

- 2 cups of almond milk,

- 1/2 cup of chia seeds, 2 tablespoons of maple syrup,
- 1 teaspoon of vanilla essence, and
- 1/2 teaspoon of cinnamon

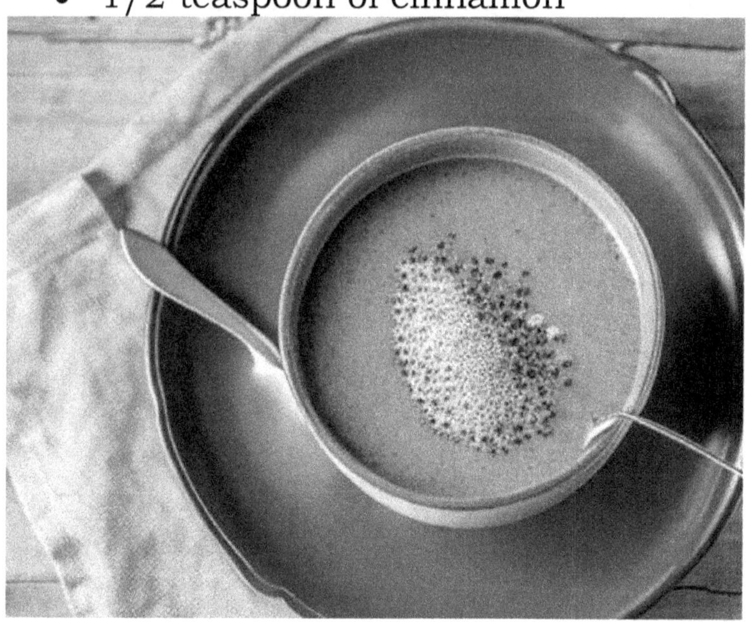

Instructions:

- To thoroughly blend the almond milk, chia seeds, maple syrup, vanilla essence, and cinnamon, stir them all together in a medium bowl.
- Protect with a lid and chill for at least 4 hours or overnight.
- Offer cold. Enjoy!

CHAPTER 5

SMOOTHIES RECIPES
Blueberry Acai Green Tea Smoothie

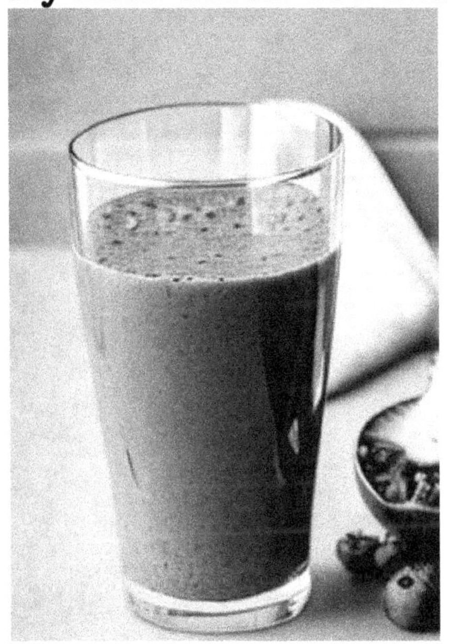

Ingredients:

- 1/4 cup Frozen blueberries; 2 tsp. Acai Powder
- 1 cup of brewed and chilled green tea
- 2 tablespoons of honey; 1 banana

Instructions:

- Blend acai powder, frozen blueberries, green tea, honey, and banana in a food processor.
- Purée until fluid.

- Dish out and savor!

Refreshing Peaches and Mango Smoothie

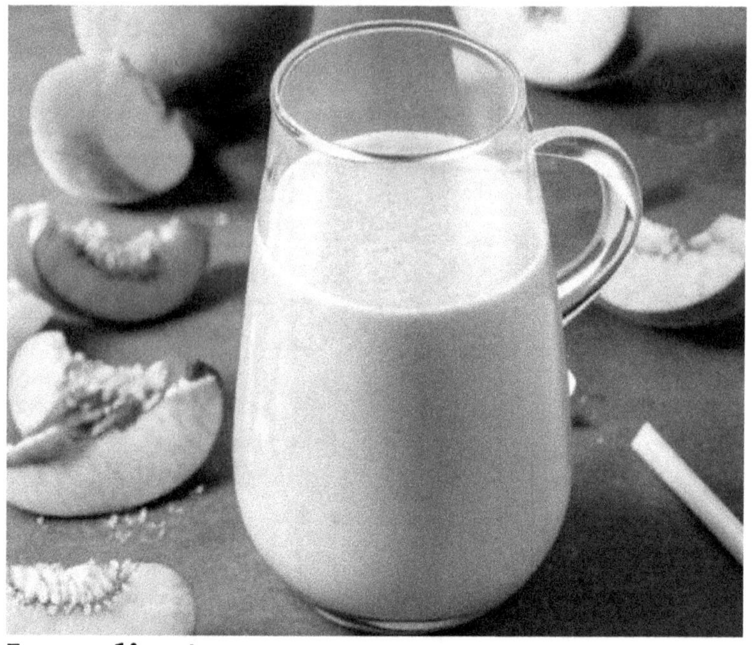

Ingredients:

- Two mangos, peeled, pitted, and cubed;
- two peaches, pitted and cut; two mango
- 2 tsp. chia seeds;
- 2 tsp. fresh mint;
- 1/2 cups of unsweetened almond milk

Instructions:

- Fill a blender with mangos, peaches, almond milk, chia seeds, and fresh mint.
- Purée until fluid.
- Dish out and savor!

Smoothie with oranges to boost immunity:

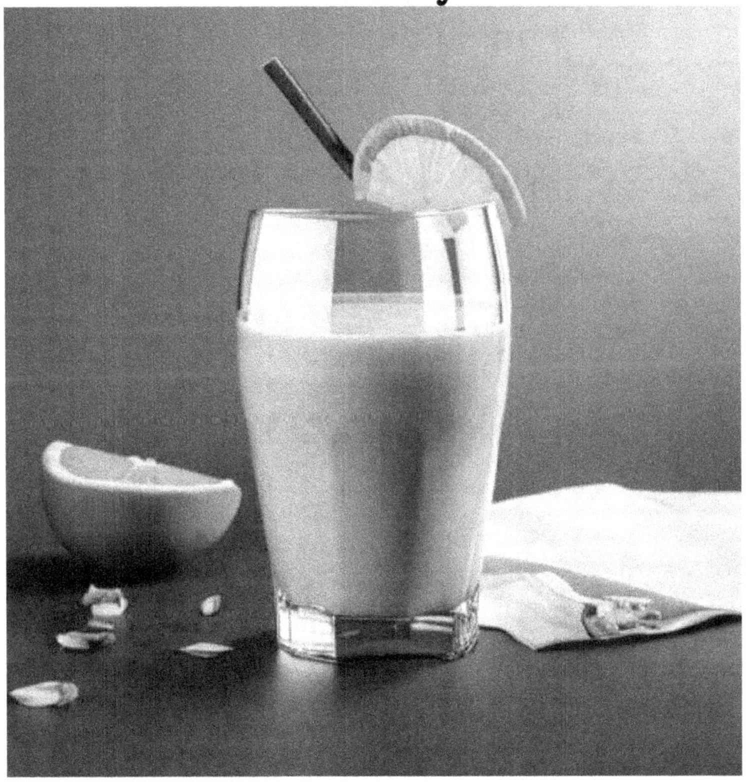

Ingredients:
- 1 cup coconut water;
- 2 oranges, peeled and segmented

- 2 cups baby spinach;
- 1 teaspoon turmeric powder
- two pitted Dates

Instructions:

- In a blender, combine oranges, baby spinach, coconut water, turmeric powder, and dates.
- Purée until fluid.
- Dish out and savor!

Smoothie with Apple And Carrot Antioxidants

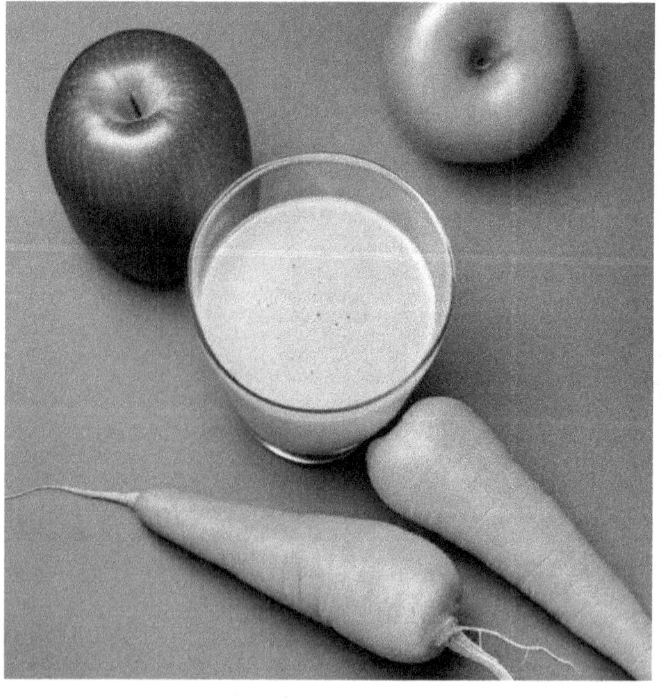

Ingredients:

- 1 peeled and cubed apple
- 2 peeled and chopped carrots
- 1 cup unsweetened almond milk
- 2 teaspoons hemp seeds
- 1/2 teaspoon Ground Cinnamon

Instructions:

- In a blender, combine the apple, the carrots, the almond milk, the hemp seeds, and the ground cinnamon.
- Purée until fluid.
- Dish out and savor!

Cherry and Dark Chocolate Smoothies

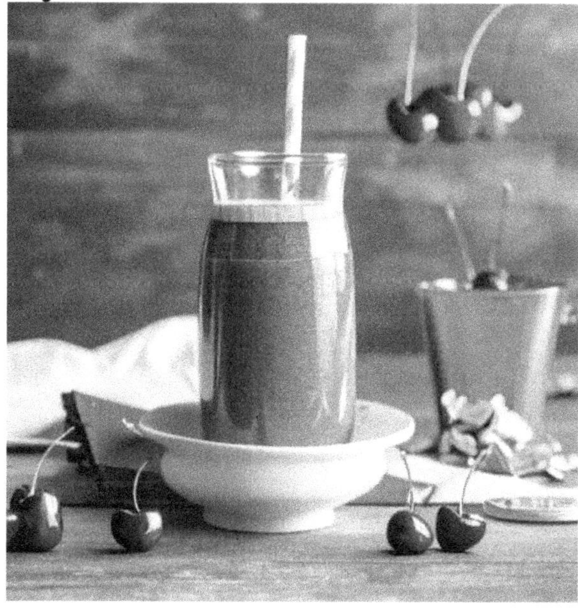

Ingredients:
- A half cup of frozen cherries
- One banana
- 2 tbsp. of unsweetened cocoa powder
- 2 tsp. of flax seeds
- One cup of almond milk

Instructions:
- In a blender, combine the cherries, banana, chocolate powder, flax seeds, and almond milk.
- Purée until fluid.
- Dish out and savor!

CHAPTER 6

MEAL PLAN

DAY ONE:
- Breakfast: Banana Nut Overnight Oats
- Lunch: Avocado Chickpea Wraps
- Dinner: Quinoa Stuffed Peppers
- Dessert: Raw Trio Bars
- Smoothie: Cherry and Dark Chocolate Smoothie

DAY TWO:
- Breakfast: Baked Mushroom and Asparagus Frittata
- Lunch: Fennel, Apple and Walnut Salad
- Dinner: Super Green Pesto Pasta
- Dessert: Vegan Matcha Cheesecake
- Smoothie: Refreshing Peaches and Mango Smoothie

DAY THREE:
- Breakfast: Avocado Toast with Roasted Tomatoes
- Lunch: Roasted Vegetable Bowls
- Dinner: Roasted Eggplant and Cashew Curry

- Dessert: Banana-Strawberry Ice Cream
- Smoothie: Immunity Boosting Orange Smoothie

DAY FOUR:

- Breakfast: Almond Butter and Jam Toast
- Lunch: Charred Cauliflower and Kale Salad
- Dinner: Broccoli and Sweet Potato Fritters
- Dessert: Coconut-Lemon Blondies
- Smoothie: Carrot and Apple Antioxidant Smoothie

DAY FIVE:

- Breakfast: Buckwheat Waffles
- Lunch: Lentil Tacos
- Dinner: Grilled Portobello Mushrooms
- Dessert: Chia Seed Pudding
- Smoothie: Blueberry Acai Green Tea Smoothie

CONCLUSION

If you're a vegan and want to lower your risk of heart disease, this book is a must-have resource. The dishes are delectable, simple to prepare, and enable readers to maintain a vegan diet while satisfying their dietary requirements. This comprehensive manual on a healthy vegan diet includes guidelines, meal-planning advice, and instructional articles. This cookbook teaches readers how to prepare delectable, heart-healthy vegan meals that will energize both their bodies and minds. This book is chock-full of insightful guidance that can lower and avoid the risk of heart discasc in vegans.

I'm grateful that you took the time to read my book. I hope you like it and it gave you something to think about. Thank You

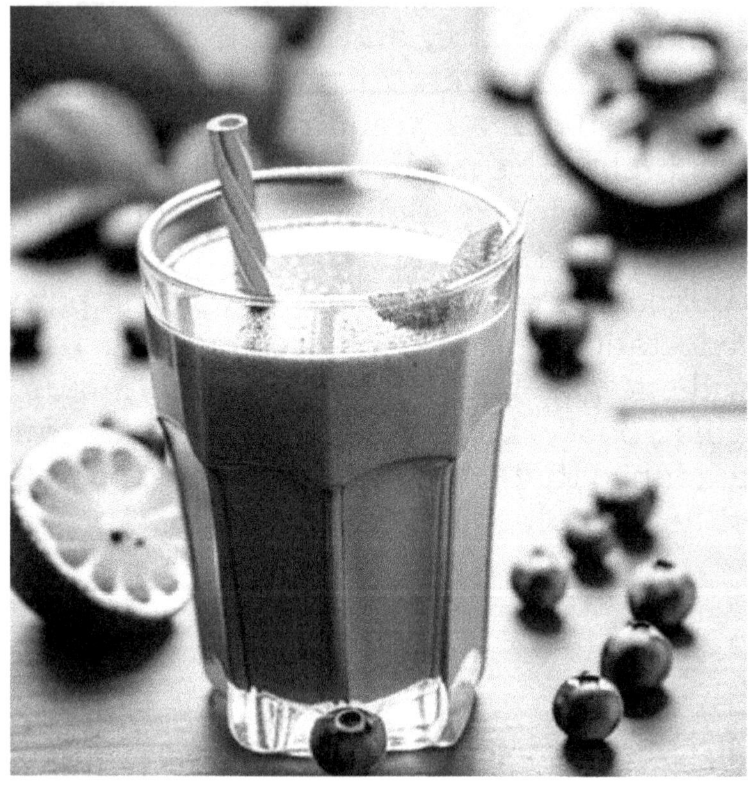

MEAL PLANNER

WEEK________

MONDAY

BREAKFAST

LUNCH

DINNER

DESSERTS

SNACKS

TUESDAY

BREAKFAST

LUNCH

DINNER

DESSERTS

SNACKS

WENESDAY

BREAKFAST

LUNCH

DINNER

DESSERTS

SNACKS

THURSDAY

BREAKFAST

LUNCH

DINNER

DESSERTS

SNACKS

FRIDAY

BREAKFAST

LUNCH

DINNER

DESSERTS

SNACKS

SATURDAY

BREAKFAST

LUNCH

DINNER

DESSERTS

SNACKS

SUNDAY

BREAKFAST

LUNCH

DINNER

DESSERTS

SNACKS

NOTES

WEEK________

MONDAY

BREAKFAST

____

____

LUNCH

____

____

DINNER

____

____

DESSERTS

____

____

SNACKS

____

____

TUESDAY

BREAKFAST

____

____

LUNCH

____

____

DINNER

____

DESSERTS

____

SNACKS

____

____

WENESDAY

BREAKFAST

____

LUNCH

____

DINNER

____

DESSERTS

____

SNACKS

THURSDAY

BREAKFAST

LUNCH

DINNER

DESSERTS

SNACKS

FRIDAY

BREAKFAST

LUNCH

DINNER

DESSERTS

SNACKS

SATURDAY

BREAKFAST

LUNCH

DINNER

DESSERTS

SNACKS

____

SUNDAY

BREAKFAST

____

LUNCH

____

DINNER

____

DESSERTS

____

SNACKS

____

NOTES

____

____

____

____

WEEK_________

MONDAY

BREAKFAST

____

____

LUNCH

____

____

DINNER

____

____

DESSERTS

____

____

SNACKS

____

____

TUESDAY

BREAKFAST

____

____

LUNCH

____

____

DINNER

____

DESSERTS

____

SNACKS

____

WENESDAY

BREAKFAST

____

LUNCH

____

DINNER

____

DESSERTS

____

SNACKS

____

THURSDAY
BREAKFAST
____

LUNCH
____

DINNER
____

DESSERTS
____

SNACKS
____

FRIDAY
BREAKFAST
____

LUNCH

DINNER

____

DESSERTS

____

SNACKS

____

SATURDAY

BREAKFAST

____

LUNCH

____

DINNER

____

DESSERTS

____

SNACKS

____

____

SUNDAY

BREAKFAST

____

____

LUNCH

____

____

DINNER

____

____

DESSERTS

____

____

SNACKS

____

____

NOTES

____

____

____

____

WEEK________

MONDAY

BREAKFAST

____

____

LUNCH

____

DINNER

____

____

DESSERTS

____

SNACKS

____

____

TUESDAY

BREAKFAST

____

____

LUNCH

____

____

DINNER

DESSERTS

SNACKS

WENESDAY

BREAKFAST

LUNCH

DINNER

DESSERTS

SNACKS

THURSDAY

BREAKFAST

LUNCH

DINNER

DESSERTS

SNACKS

FRIDAY

BREAKFAST

LUNCH

DINNER

DESSERTS

SNACKS

SATURDAY

BREAKFAST

LUNCH

DINNER

DESSERTS

SUNDAY

BREAKFAST

LUNCH

DINNER

DESSERTS

SNACKS

NOTES